Sixty Five and Still Alive?

MESOTHELIOMA

By Pete O'Connell

From 2007 -2011

Sixty Five and Still Alive?

Preface

This book is intended to let you take a look at my experiences in dealing with a terminal illness, from diagnosis in July 2007 through surgery, radiotherapy, chemotherapy and complimentary therapies and up to my sixty fifth birthday (?) in January 2012.

*It will look at my battles with myself and the medics and looking at the other options open to people with cancer. I also wish this book to be used to encourage anyone with **Mesothelioma** to live and to become a survivor not a victim of this evil disease.*

And to come each day to realise.

Yesterday is history.

Tomorrow is unknown.

So live each day as best you can.

Measure your progress by week not by day.

And remember; only your God knows when you will die.

Sixty Five and Still Alive?

Dedications

To my family and friends who have helped me be a survivor rather than a victim.

But especially to Yvonne my rock and my source of strength throughout this whole dreadful part of my life she has been my reason to stay alive. Yvonne signed up for 20/30yr life with an older man who was fit, successful and came from a family with great longevity, but after seven years she had inherited a terminally ill man of 60 years with 6 months to two years to live (or so the Medics have said).

Yvonne, without you I would have given up and would not be around to write this book.

It would be wrong not to mention the help from the medical fraternity who in many ways have helped me survive, Jo Hamilton, Frank Collins and his team, my GP and especially Professor Lewis for the positive and supportive way he has dealt with me.

I would also like to recognise the 30 years I spent with my first wife Val who like Yvonne gave me love, loyalty and support in everything I did.

I wish all profits from this book to go to Macmillan Cancer Support and Cancer Research for the continuing investigation into Mesothelioma and how to cure and support this dreadful disease.

Sixty Five and Still Alive?

CONTENTS

Sixty Five and Still Alive?

CHAPTER ONE

LIFE BEFORE CANCER

My story begins in early December 1999, at 52 years old, I had been happily married to Val for 31 years, with two grown up children Kay and Neil and one grandchild Courtney. I had just been appointed as Head of Operations at work and had assumed responsibility for a turnover of £40 million per year and a work force of around 350 people mostly home-based auditors spread across the UK and Europe.

In mid-December of 1999 my life was thrown into turmoil when I fell in love with Yvonne "the love of my life" and my wonderful wife, this was not a relationship I had sort nor was it something I had wanted or expected and I do not want to spend time or print on justification or to gather support or sympathy for the event, but it happened and I have no regrets.

We have been together since August 2000, she is my rock and my anchor and without her I would not be around to write this book. Yvonne came with two children from her previous marriage, Michelle, 12 and Ella, 9.

Our first few months were fraught with problems two unpleasant divorces and social services giving custody of two little girls to a smoking, drinking, womanising wife beater because he lived nearer to the school they had been attending, this situation did not last too long as Ella, the little one, was missing her mum and after two weeks came to live with us regardless of the social services stupidity. Sadly, the elder one Michelle stayed put and had been estranged from her mum for most of her teenage years, however she is now 23 and doing a PhD in Sheffield and they are thankfully much closer now.

We married in March 2002 by which time we had gained a new grandchild Rebekah, so with four kids and two grandkids we set out on married life like many people as enthusiastic restarts with readymade families.

I had been a very healthy man with loads of energy and a successful career and at 52 years old felt I could offer Yvonne 30 years or so together. In 2003 I took the decision to start our own business in consultancy and after many years working for large organisations, I felt it was time to try living on my own

Sixty Five and Still Alive?

ability. Over a two-year period, we opened two companies and started employing staff; Yvonne joined the companies in 2006 making us a true family business. All was going well, however I did contract Pneumonia in May 2005 and spent 2 months feeling really unwell.

The businesses continued to grow and by 2007 we were turning over around £500,000 per year. All was well and life was good; a great life, a successful set of businesses and a bright future with a turnover of one million forecasted for 2007/2008.

Since we got married in 2002: Kay had married her kid's dad in 2003, Yvonne and I had rebuilt our new home in Bromsgrove (a 1964 bungalow) and we had both worked our socks off rebuilding my sons house in Dudley in 2005, so that he could go off to Brighton with his girlfriend to start an Internet business. So, I was certainly OK at this stage. Then in January 2007 we went to Vegas, Hawaii, and San Francisco for my sixtieth birthday and yes, I did walk up that famous big hill in San Francisco.

In the middle of July of 2007, we went to Cyprus for a family wedding, during the one week break I felt quite breathless and unwell. On return to the UK I felt like I had contracted Pneumonia again, a visit to the doctors had me despatched to the local hospital, it was not Pneumonia, it was, I was told an infection in the lining of the right lung that could be removed by micro surgery. My operation took place on the 1st August 2007. A 12-inch scar and 5 hours in surgery was not what I had expected in conjunction with the phrase 'micro' but when the doctor looked at me in the recovery room and said, it was very messy but he had not seen anything sinister, but to be safe he had sent samples to histology for confirmation, I felt quite positive for the future.

After a problem of post-operative oedema (swelling up like a Michelin man) something you can laugh about but you don't want it to happen to you, I left the hospital on the 10th August feeling lucky to be OK and now looking forward to getting back to work. During my time in the hospital I had become friends with a guy called Chris who helped me during my early post-operative days. Chris had had two lobes of his right lung removed from lung cancer and at this stage I used to think how lucky I was to have had a mere infection. In fact, I remember running across a car park in Birmingham and Chris asking me to slow down as he could not keep up.

Sixty Five and Still Alive?

On the 1st September I was back at work and starting to feel well and in control of my life again. I remember my first job being at Plymouth Hospital and finding it difficult to site the caravan but I was coping and I was able to get on with things. A visit to the specialist chest clinic in Birmingham to see the head surgeon on the 14th September confirmed this, I was told I was fine and had probably had pollen particles or a foreign body invade my lung lining. Wonderful, I was going to be OK, the luck of the Irish holding good.

Yvonne was with me as she always is (this will become my catch phrase) and asked what the histology report had said, "Oh" said the surgeon "it does not appear to be in the file but I am sure it will be ok and we will be in contact with you soon".

Sixty Five and Still Alive?

CHAPTER TWO

THE NEWS AND PROGNOSIS

Good news in September at the Birmingham chest clinic.

To despair and disbelief in October.

I returned home from work on the 16th October 2007 to an answer phone message asking me to attend an appointment at the Alexandra Hospital the following day with the thoracic department. I convinced myself it was to be discharged from the Hospital, how wrong I was.

I was greeted by the Dr and a Macmillan nurse, as always Yvonne was at my side, "I have some bad news for you" said the doctor, "you have mesothelioma".

"I have what?" I asked.

"Mesothelioma caused by asbestos" replied the doctor.

I asked what the prognosis was. I have no idea why I asked for the prognosis as I have never worked or played with asbestos and after the first few sentences from the doctor; I had not heard anything that was said. But Yvonne and I are auditors and consultants we write everything down. Sad, but that's just the way we are (a habit that has been very helpful over the years and has given us the whole of chapter eight). Sad, but true.

"You have maybe six months to a year" he said, "and if you are very lucky two years".

"But I feel so well", I retorted.

"Well that is because you have had an operation" he said, "but it will all come back, I am sorry, but it will. If we had known what it was, we would not have operated".

He then spent a long time telling me I could claim damages for an industrial injury and I should get a solicitor and contact the DWP; most of this was not

Sixty Five and Still Alive?

sinking in; I hope this was not the prescribed method of telling people they are going to die.

My rock was in tears, not something I had seen before, she is a very strong lady who does not show emotion in the way I do (I can cry for England). But Yvonne cares very deeply and is not prone to the dramatic.

Then the doctor said, "and you will need radiotherapy to the scar to stop the tumour breaking out through the tissue, it will make you more comfortable, so I will refer you to an Oncologist". (*What on earth had I got*, was how that made me think).

With that, we left the hospital. I was supposed to be going to Manchester to do a half day job and I said to Yvonne "I will drop you at home and get off to the job then!" Of course, I did not go to Manchester I was stopped by the boss.

When we got home Yvonne's dad was staying with us. At that time, he was eighty-six quite frail and struggling to reach the pan. We explained our meeting with the doctor and why we were both a little distressed, he waited till he and I were on our own and then said to me "I will come and look after her for you when you have gone."

That struck home more than anything the doctor had said, my wife was going to be comforted and looked after by an old man who needed constant support himself, I was in bits, but god bless you Albert for the kind offer. Sadly, Albert died in May 2011 so would have been unable to carry out the task, but I am sure he would have tried his best had the opportunity been available.

Telling family and friends is not easy; most people need to be told more than once, as they keep saying things to you like "are you sure!" "what did you say?" "you're joking." Well I can tell you, joker I am, but not with this situation. The more people ask the less competent you become at getting the mouth to say the correct thing, so writing it down is not a bad idea and to say "I am going to die" was impossible.

My daughter Kay took the news very badly. We are very close and speak on the phone daily, she had not been impressed when I had got divorced but over time has come to terms with how life is. She had been constantly at the hospital during my illness which was an achievement while looking after two youngsters and a husband when the hospital is 20 miles away from her home.

Sixty Five and Still Alive?

My son was also horrified at the news but living 130 miles from me he was unable to spend the same amount of time visiting us but has been coming to the West Midlands as and when it has been possible.

As the only child of two only children I have no close relatives of my own, other than my two kids, but I do have a great bunch of relatives inherited from two wives, both of whom come from large families and believe me they have all been brilliant and have helped me a lot over the years, but particularly Yvonne's younger sister, Marie and her wonderful kids. Who have consistently shown concern and compassion and perhaps most of all for their prayers and belief in divine intervention.

Then there is Fred (my first wife's brother) who is always on hand and ready to come round and baby sit me or go out for lunch. So the saying you can pick your friends but you inherit your relatives has been good for me and flies in the face of the saying, as the inherited relatives are, in most, better than the friends I have picked and when you have a terminal illness you soon find who wants to keep in touch and who wants out, even sadly out of thirty year friendships.

I spoke once in the Oncology unit at Redditch to a couple who set off on a world cruise saying goodbye to all the people they had met that had impacted on them after being given the news of a terminal illness. I have had no such desire to do this type of thing.

The day after my death sentence was pronounced, I went to see my GP; what a difference from the blunt and callas Thoracic department. He was attentive compassionate and has continued since that day to be a credit to the medical fraternity. He has even rung me late evenings to reassure me and to check I am OK (good on you Doc).

Very soon an appointment came through to see an Oncologist, a Doctor Jo Hamilton at the Alexandra Hospital on the 7th November 2007.

Jo Hamilton has now been my Oncologist for several years, she is a young woman with very fixed ideas but does listen to me and has on occasions done what I have asked, she has a nice bed side manner and has also helped me to survive.

However, the meeting on the 7th November 2007 was my first encounter with Dr Hamilton, she explained that anything she could do must be regarded as Palliative (incurable and for comfort only) and that radiotherapy to the scar

Sixty Five and Still Alive?

tissue was normal and would help to stop any spread of the tumour to the outside of my body. The second time this had been mentioned and a little worrying. She explained that left untreated, the tumour mass can track down the scar line and form very uncomfortable and painful lumps, luckily the treatment must have worked as I have had no problem in this area, and it is now 2011. The secondary bone cancer, I developed later, is proof of the ferocity of the tumours and became a real problem with my shoulder in 2011.

I attended a planning meeting at Coventry's Walsgrave Hospital on the 15th November 2007; the treatment was to be 16 gray over two fractions of 6mv, starting on the 29th November and ending a week later on the 6th December.

I am showing off a little here because as a consultancy business I have spent a lot of time auditing departments in the NHS and in private hospitals: I have a good understanding of oncology and had also let Jo Hamilton know I was quite clued up.

The story of my life has always been a lucky one but I don't do things the easy way as this book will make clear and on turning up for my first fraction of radiotherapy I was told the applicator was distorted due to being left on the windowsill and I would have to make a new appointment! I told them to pack it with bolus which prompted a very strange look from the radiographer and her team. A few minutes later Jo Hamilton arrived looked at the applicator then looked at me and said "I think you should do what he says," she then stroked my arm and said "you know it may make you a little red," "yes" I said "but just flipping do it."

I had questioned the diagnosis with the thoracic guy and had asked to see the surgical team as the comment "nothing sinister" was haunting me from the August debrief with the surgeon. An appointment had been arranged by the Thoracic's Doctor for the 16th November at the Birmingham chest clinic.

I met the registrar on the 16th and found the meeting encouraging; he confirmed that the whole plural lining had been removed during surgery and that if the tumour returned it could be de-bulked (yuck). He also said if it had been known that the problem was mesothelioma he would still have carried out the same operation and that what had been done was the best option.

I was at this stage still not convinced that the diagnosis was mine and as I felt quite well, I kept saying to Yvonne they have got it wrong.

Sixty Five and Still Alive?

CHAPTER THREE

HOW TO BECOME VERY RICH FROM A DEATH SENTENCE (UNLESS YOUR NAME IS O'CONNELL)

I had been told that Mesothelioma was an industrial issue that you could claim vast sums of money from previous employers and that the DWP would also make payments against an Industrial Injuries Claim. I had to find a solicitor who was proficient in this type of claim. We eventually selected Thompsons and in particular a guy called Terry Loughery, his first visit to us was on the 23 October 2007, a very clued up man used to this type of claim and well versed in Mesothelioma.

I could be claiming around £50,000 - £70,000 for pain and suffering and £500,000 for loss of income plus nursing care and other incidentals, a cool £600,000 not worth dying for, but wow, better than nothing.

We spent a few hours going over my childhood, schooling, work history and any other relevant trips to try and establish how I had contracted the illness. Now with every person he has dealt with in the past, establishing the source of the exposure had been easy, they had been a plumber, a mechanic, a ship builder etc. But me, I am a pen pusher. After much deliberation I had convinced myself that the exposure had come from an asbestos roof in a building I had worked in some 40 years earlier. Terry was pleased that we had arrived at a source of infection and had said he would arrange for me to see a guy called Professor Sherwood Burge for a consultation, and for him to become our medical expert during court cases and negotiations with the employer.

We completed an insurance document that covered the costs of the legal and medical bills and Terry left assuring me all was well. During this afternoon of fun, he had said he may not be able to finish the case before I died but he would ensure Yvonne did not lose out, when I explained to him that I did not believe the diagnosis he gave me a strange and telling look that said "poor pratt."

We had several phone conversations during the weeks that followed and on the 3rd January 2008, I went to see Professor Sherwood Burge at the Birmingham chest clinic, he carried out functional lung tests and then spent two hours going over my life, from birth to current times.   He said he thought I was very well

Sixty Five and Still Alive?

for a man with Mesothelioma (more support for my "they got it wrong theory") and he said he would personally check the histology reports and speak to the surgical team.

After some weeks a note arrived from Professor Burge. It just said, "sorry, I would confirm having checked the histology data, that you have Mesothelioma."

After months of phone calls and a couple of visits from Terry Loughery of Thompsons it was decided that I had no one to claim off and that the asbestos roof I had identified from my youth had been demolished in around 1990 but was probably steel or tin and because the employer was a micro business we had no chance of winning a case in the courts. The luck of the Irish again the only terminally ill man in the world who has no recourse and no one to claim off! So, by the 12th Feb 2008 any thought of money for death had been discounted.

Terry rang me some weeks later and asked if I was prepared for him to submit a claim to an American legal company who were handling asbestos claims for a South African or American importer of asbestos in to the UK in the 60s and 70s, this produced a cheque for £4k not the £600k I had been told but better than nothing.

As mentioned earlier the DWP regard this illness as an industrial injury so we had made a claim for compensation from the state, which is assessed on age and other criteria. Again, I know people who have received significantly more than we were paid, but never the less I did have a cheque for around £30,000 that I promptly added a few grand to and spent it on a second hand Jaguar XKR convertible, a wonderful car that makes me feel good. I had thought of having a note on the number plate saying "partly funded by the DWP" but on reflection, decided it may not be one of my better ideas.

On the 12th February 2008 the DWP sent a lovely lady to see me she wanted to help me with all sorts of things, she spent an hour or so going through the things I might be able to claim for.

"Do you need help undressing?" she said; "only if we are going to have sex" I said!

Sixty Five and Still Alive?

"How do you manage with bathing?" and so on, she kept this up for ages, but nothing was of much use to me as I was quite fit and well at this stage and was still on the "I am ok" phase.

She did however assist me in getting a disabled badge and free road tax for my car (not the XKR). This has proven very helpful over the years and saved me lots of time and money (well done that lady).

Sixty Five and Still Alive?

CHAPTER FOUR

SLASH BURN AND POISON OR WHAT DOCTORS CALL ONCOLOGY

I have mentioned previously my involvement in oncology has been professional as well as being on the receiving end. I have audited most of the country's leading cancer units, Christies, The Royal Marsden, The QE, St James Leeds, Derricot, Bristol & Bath. The list is very long and I have been privileged to meet and talk to some of the country's leading cancer specialists.

I have at the time of writing this chapter had surgery (Slash) in August 2007 and, three doses of Radiotherapy (Burn) in Dec 2007, June 2010 and August 2010 and I am part way through my second cycle of chemotherapy treatment (Poison) in September 2010.

Like most Cancers, Mesothelioma is treated with all three available treatment options, often surgery is not an option due to late detection and oncologists are left with only the chemotherapy or radiotherapy options.

At the time of my diagnosis in 2007 Alimta was not available in this Country (Licenced by N I C E as No 35 in January 2008 for use in the UK). I am told other drugs did not work well with these tumours, so surgery and radiotherapy were the front-line treatments.

Having experienced the three main cancer treatments, I can say without any doubt that chemotherapy is the most horrendous experience I have ever had in my life, but for me it is the treatment that works the best, I am writing this chapter with my nose bleeding profusely from a significant drop in my platelet count and feeling washed out due to a drop in the red blood cells, will I do it again? Well you bet, I intend to continue with my life for as long as God and the medics are prepared to help me survive and I firmly believe that we are all entitled to see three score year and 10 "the old biblical 70 years a man's life expectancy".

To achieve this though I need to continue to live for a further six years and three months!! Or in mesothelioma speak, six times longer than the average person lives from diagnosis to death; on top of the 3.5 years I have already survived, but as an Iranian Medical Scientist friend of mine Hajie told me in 2007 "Peter

Sixty Five and Still Alive?

only your God knows when you will die". So, we will have to see what happens.

Now I have a really good friendship with a guy called Vic who has the same disease as me, he was diagnosed in December 2009 and has had slash and poison as a continuous flow, operation in January 2010 and Chemotherapy during March, April and May 2010. The surgery Vic had was a little more radical than mine with the surgeon removing the lung lining, the sac from the heart and part of his lung; this is now an alternative operation from the one performed by David Waller (one of the pioneers of mesothelioma treatments,) who removes the infected lung, a large part of the diaphragm and the sacs from the stomach and heart.

I met Vic through speaking to his wife Heather on a Facebook Meso site and we are now good friends, it will be interesting to see how his disease develops over the coming years and be able to compare the two treatments for effectiveness.

I had an operation for an unknown lung complaint on the 1st August 2007, one dose of Radiotherapy to the scar tissue in December 2007 and then went 20 months without any treatment and then went onto chemotherapy as a last chance saloon in March 2009. I would think that the treatment Vic has had will give him a much better start than I had, but time will tell.

Cancer treatment is evolving all the time and new treatments are being trialled and released almost weekly. During my limited time auditing oncology units, I have seen the introduction of Prostrate Brach therapy, advances in nuclear medicines and the use of cryo techniques.

Sadly, mesothelioma is a rare cancer and I don't think much research or investment goes in to finding answers and a cure. It is one of a handful of cancers that are described as incurable and only treatable in a palliative way.

I hope this book is capable of making a small contribution to assist in funding research into this dreadful and debilitating nightmare of a disease and that oncologists continue to encourage people to fight and survive the effects of this disease.

Sixty Five and Still Alive?

CHAPTER FIVE

THE OSTRICH YEAR

In January 2008 I had an appointment come through to see Jo Hamilton Consultant Oncologist at the Alexandra hospital Redditch. I had seen the surgical registrar in November, met with Professor Sherwood Burge in January 2008 and the X-rays in November and January had shown that no further reduction was taking place in the lung function. Once the lining has been removed the lung attaches itself to the side of the rib cage so does not give a fully functioning organ and your breathing is never going to be 100% but I had 66% of my lung capacity and as we only use around 30% for normal activities I felt fine, I think the expression used was only a marathon would use full function.

I told Jo Hamilton on the 15th January 2008 that I would contact her as and when I felt unwell, she agreed to this but insisted that I go and see her if things changed. As I walked through the Alexandra Hospital from Jo's consulting room I said to Yvonne "well, we will see her in 10 years then".

So started the Ostrich year, I was well, we booked a holiday to Cuba for the end of January to continue my love affair with a county I had become obsessed with 10 years earlier, we had a great time and returned home in early February. I was working five days a week and enjoying life; as the weeks went by I was convinced that the diagnosis was wrong, though with hindsight I was not breathing as well as I should and had started to call it panic attacks and over breathing. I was working in St James Hospital in Leeds in the spring of 2008 and had mentioned my situation to the senior radiographer; she said to me "Oh you have adopted the Ostrich approach, have you?" "Yes" I said.

As the months went by I was getting more breathless but it wasn't cancer it was being unfit, it was a chest infection or I was over breathing. Clearly I was mad not to see what was happening but I continued to go on holidays to the Caribbean on a cruise and to lots of weekend breaks. I did however use the condition if it was to my advantage! Like in March 2008 at a weekend break for our wedding anniversary when the accommodation and the hotel were less than good. I told the receptionist I was terminally ill and they had screwed up what

Sixty Five and Still Alive?

would be my last anniversary celebration with my wife. I had previously, when shopping for a Christmas present in the December of 2007, needed a new watch and was being pushed by the sales assistant in the jewellers to take out a three-year warranty. "I don't want a three-year warranty I only have a few months left to live" I said. She was mortified and broke in to tears, Yvonne said I was a rotten sod to do that to her, the watch is over three years old now and I am still here, so I saved the cost of additional warranty but I don't do that type of thing anymore. Well not too often and only if I am in the mood.

I had taken out a disabled badge after the visit by the DWP lady and will now admit that without it; I would have really struggled at the back end of 2008 as my breathing and walking were dreadful. Christmas came and went we had a few parties and spent time with family and friends so as 2009 began I was working 5 days a week and travelling all over the country again.

In January 2009 we went to the Gran Canaries for a week in a very posh hotel with a room on the 3rd floor. On arrival I felt really unwell, I have a chest infection; I told Yvonne. I had been ill since Christmas and had struggled to walk up a flight of stairs in early January, but my daughter Kay was getting married again in the March and I was not prepared to admit I had a problem and be laid up in hospital. I spent the whole week in the bedroom of the hotel and had to be put on the plane home by a disabled lift to the side of the plane, I had seen a doctor while on holiday who had prescribed antibiotics and other potions and pills.

Once home I went to my own GP who said, "you need to go to hospital". I was admitted to the Alexandra on the 3rd February 2009. I had gone a year without seeing any one, but I had been very foolish and will not be doing that again. The X-ray shows the lack of the right lung in March 2009; the document below covers the over breathing I had convinced myself I was doing.

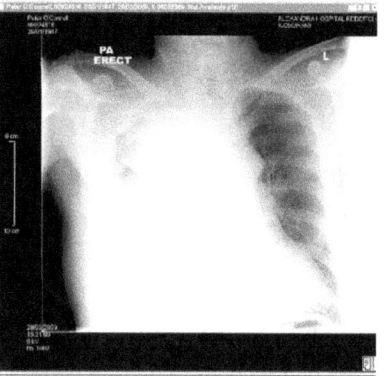

Sixty Five and Still Alive?

OVERBREATHING

Over breathing (medical name 'hyperventilation') means a habit of breathing incorrectly and excessively. It can result from emotional stress and can cause tension or anxiety. Over breathing upsets the chemistry of the body and can lead to many physical and emotional symptoms. Frequent sighing, yawning or swallowing air can add to the problem.

SYMPTOMS

Dizziness, lightheaded, feeling faint; headaches; tension in your head; being easily tired; ringing in the ears; blurred vision; dry mouth; hard to swallow; sweating; shortness of breath; heart beating faster; palpitations; shaking hands; numbness or tingling of hands, feet or face; aches and pains in your limbs; bloated stomach; nausea; diarrhea; passing wind up or down; apprehension; tension; agitation.

You can learn better breathing habits which will reduce many of these symptoms. However, it is not always easy to change habits and it may take some time. The actions outlined below have been useful to other people with this problem.

Sixty Five and Still Alive?

TREATMENT

Step 1   Breath as slowly as you can using your stomach and not your chest. If possible, breathe only through your nose; in while counting 5 to yourself and then out while counting 5 to yourself

Step 2   Sit or lie in a quiet place where you will not be interrupted and breathe like this for 5 minutes several times a day. Most people find this uncomfortable at first until the body is used to it.

Step 3   When you can do this easily then lengthen the time spent each day. Start to practice slow breathing when sitting quietly, for example watching TV or on a bus. Practice by speaking more slowly or by reading out loud.

Step 4   Eventually you will be able to breathe slowly all the time unless upset or frightened by something. Prepare for such times by breathing slowly beforehand and afterwards.

Blocked breathing   Another method is to take a breath, hold your nose with your mouth closed and push your breath as if you are trying to breathe out or are 'popping' your ears. Blocking your breathing in this way will calm your heart and your breathing within a few moments.

Re-breathing   If you find it difficult to start the above exercises or if you cannot control your breathing in certain situations, hold a paper bag (big enough for a loaf of bread) over your mouth and nose. Breathe as deeply as you like but only breathe the air inside the bag. You will begin to feel better after a few minutes of this (it is not safe to use a plastic bag).

Sixty Five and Still Alive?

SIGHING, YAWNING OR SWALLONING AIR

If you become aware of any of these habits, try to take a single ordinary breath instead or hold your breath for five seconds.

Relaxation, yoga, tai chi or meditation may also help you to slow your breathing.

This does work and I can recommend it for relaxation.

I believe you need three things to be a survivor.

1) You need to have enormous determination to survive as some of the treatments are dreadful and at times you want to be dead.
2) You need medical assistance whatever that may be.
3) You need the third dimension call it divine intervention, what will be will be or luck. Without this element survival is even harder. I had a discussion on this subject with a guy at the chemo clinic a week or so ago, he thinks I am mad and said it is all to do with the ferocity of the disease. I would beg to differ and after an interesting hour or so we agreed to disagree. You must make up your own minds, (as I have found nothing is as it seems).

Sixty Five and Still Alive?

CHAPTER SIX

LIFE GOES ON IN DOWNTOWN BROMSGROVE

In January 2011 I had to accept that the secondary bone cancer that had developed and was found in my right arm back in July 2010, was gaining ground and making me feel really ill; it is very painful with few avenues open to you other than pain killers and radiotherapy. After a broken arm, and radiotherapy to my spine on two other occasions; I now had a large golf ball sized lump on my left shoulder where the cancer (Mesothelioma) had broken out through the site of the arm operation from July 2010. In April 2011 I had been told again the end of the road was coming and that chemotherapy and radiotherapy were becoming less of an option; as they made me very ill and the oncologist was not prepared to help or contribute to my death by prescribing drugs that she was unhappy with.

I had spoken to our local hospice "The Primrose Centre" at the suggestion of the Macmillan nurse, who said it may be of some interest to me. I agreed to do a short reflexology course and had said I was continuing with Reiki. A friend of ours is a Reiki practitioner, who had mentioned the treatment on several occasions but I had not perused it. So, with an open mind I had now decided to give it a go.

So, the man of science moves on to complimentary therapies.

Reiki is hard to explain it makes me relax, it has an effect on me and it removes pain from my bones, I can feel a great sense of heat and power transmitting from my therapist who seems to be able to know where the problems and pain are.

As I said at the start of this chapter, in theory Reiki and Science are probably not compatible *(you must make up your own minds)* I am now several weeks in to the Reiki treatment and will continue with my twice a week sessions as a positive alternative to standard treatments. I have currently had one session of

Sixty Five and Still Alive?

reflexology, but I was now back in the Alexandra hospital with a lot of pain from the left shoulder, just about a year after having it pinned and screwed.

On arrival and assessment by the triage team it had been decided to admit me for observation and treatment. Once on the ward significant swelling had taken place to the whole of my left arm and hand. I was sent for an MRI scan that had been arranged as outpatient's treatment but now covered as part of my stay. I was unable to have the scan because of discomfort and pain so it was left, I don't understand why it was left.

Once home I arranged to have the Reiki sessions again and will continue with them for the foreseeable future.

So, with complimentary therapies, what are they and what do they do?

REIKI

THE WORD REIKI IS MADE OF TWO JAPANESE WORDS - REI WHICH MEANS "GOD'S WISDOM OR THE HIGHER POWER" AND KI WHICH IS "LIFE FORCE ENERGY". SO, REIKI IS ACTUALLY "SPIRITUALLY GUIDED LIFE FORCE ENERGY."

A treatment feels like a wonderful glowing radiance that flows through and around you. Reiki treats the whole person including body, emotions, mind and spirit creating many beneficial effects that include relaxation and feelings of peace, security and wellbeing. Many have reported miraculous results.

Reiki is a simple, natural and safe method of spiritual healing and self-improvement that everyone can use. It has been effective in helping virtually every known illness and malady and always creates a beneficial effect. It also works in conjunction with all other medical or therapeutic techniques to relieve side effects and promote recovery.

An amazingly simple technique to learn, the ability to use Reiki is not taught in the usual sense but is transferred to the student during a Reiki class. This ability is passed on during an "attunement" given by a Reiki master and allows the student to tap into an unlimited supply of "life force energy" to improve one's health and enhance the quality of life.

Sixty Five and Still Alive?

Its use is not dependent on one's intellectual capacity or spiritual development and therefore is available to everyone. It has been successfully taught to thousands of people of all ages and backgrounds.

While Reiki is spiritual in nature, it is not a religion. It has no dogma, and there is nothing you must believe in order to learn and use Reiki. In fact, Reiki is not dependent on belief at all and will work whether you believe in it or not. Because Reiki comes from God, many people find that using Reiki puts them more in touch with the experience of their religion rather than having only an intellectual concept of it.

REFLEXOLOGY

Reflexology is the practice of applying pressure to the feet and hands utilizing specific thumb, finger and hand techniques without the use of oil, cream or lotion based on a system of zones and reflex areas that reflect an image of the body on the feet and hands with a premise that such work effects a physical change in the body.

Reflexology charts

A reflexology chart mirrors a reflection of the body on the feet and hands, left foot or hand representing the body's left half and right foot or hand its right half. In reflexology practice, technique is applied to the relevant reflex area(s) to prompt a change in the related part of the body. Research has demonstrated such effects for several reflex areas and their reflected parts of the body, i.e. the kidney reflex areas and the kidneys; the intestine reflex areas and the intestines and the brain reflex area and the brain.

Sixty Five and Still Alive?

ACUPUNCTURE

Acupuncture originated in China, although it has also been used in other East Asian countries. Evidence suggests that it was practiced as long as 2,000 years ago, although supporters of it often claim that it has been used for over 5,000 years. It has been intertwined with spiritual and religious practices throughout Chinese history. Acupuncture has a close association with Taoism, taoists being pioneers of the belief in body-mind-spirit consciousness.

Early accounts of acupuncture written by missionaries describe acupuncture as being quite different to what we're led to believe. The needles were large, inserted deeply and used in short duration; '30 respirations' being quoted by missionary Wilhelm Ten Rhijn in 1680. Nor is there any mention of Qi, meridians, or specific acupuncture points. These concepts were actually introduced in the 20th century, notably by Georges Soulié de Mirant in his 1939 book *L'Acupuncture Chinoise*. Before the 20th century, needles were simply inserted at the site of the pain or problem.

Surprisingly, acupuncture was not introduced into Europe until the early 18th century when it was embraced by some French physicians. They were accused of *"resurrecting an absurd doctrine from well-deserved oblivion"* by many prominent doctors however. It was not introduced into England until 1821 when it was used by midwife Edward Joukes.

The three mentioned above are probably the best known and most commonly used but a whole raft of complimentary therapies are available, I would recommend research and try them if you feel they may help you, I have now upped my Reiki sessions to 5 a week and for me they are effective.

Sixty Five and Still Alive?

CHAPTER SEVEN

THE REALITY OF WHAT YOU HAVE WRONG WITH YOU

This is an interesting thought because I have been told for four years that I had only a few months left and that I should prepare for death.

During this time, I have never felt that the end was near; in fact, at times I could forget that I had a problem and carry on as normal. Since diagnosis in 2007 I have refurbished the en-suite in the guest room, rebuilt the gazebo over the hot tub 3 times and carried out numerous DIY tasks around the house and garden. In November 2010 I undertook some very ambitious plans to relocate the office into a bedroom, build a large bedroom with en-suite in what was the office and to change the rear access to the property.

Sadly, on this occasion I had taken on more than I could cope with and this was the first time since 2007 I had been faced with the inability to finish what I had started.

To address this problem Yvonne has been on my intensive DIY courses, I have taught her to lay wooden floors and carpets, box in pipes and general wood working techniques, wallpapering and tiling. All of which are earning her brownie badges and making her uniform look very impressive. Joking apart I am now very restricted in what I can and can't do and am reduced to looking back on all the brilliant holidays and cruises we have done in the last four years, my love affair with Cuba, the Queen Mary from New York to Southampton, our time on Independence of the Seas and then all the brilliant caravan breaks we have spent together and not forgetting the wedding anniversaries and birthday breaks Yvonne and I have shared.

It is now July 2011 and four years since my cancer was diagnosed, on the 1st August 2007; Yvonne and I do not agree on this date as I had the operation in August, but it was October before I saw the results of the histology records.

I was told two weeks ago that the advancing cancer had invaded the lymphatic system and that I was looking at my life ending in 2/3 months. For the first time in four years, I believe this diagnosis to be realistic, but I haven't given up yet and with effective pain control I will solder on. But as I write this chapter, I

Sixty Five and Still Alive?

would be happy to trade the next few months for an early death, as the pain is relentless and I am unable to get up anymore, spending distressing days and nights in bed. If I am immobile, I am unhappy. Now I have taken to sending messages to Yvonne as speaking is too difficult. Example below from July 2011.

Yvonne,

I need to speak to you, but I can't, my throat is clogged up and I also get very emotional.

I think you know this, but I will try to explain what is happening to me.

1) Each day I am getting weaker and I now have trouble standing up I manage the loo, but I am very wobbly and standing up is becoming an issue, could you ask Ellen to get a raised loo seat like Ken had after his hip op.

2) I have tried to shake off the advancing weakness the rapid progress of the cancer, but this time it's not happening, and I don't want to fall over and damage any more bones so I am going to stay in bed. My left arm is unusable and very painful whether a compression bandage would help is a question for Ellen.

3) I have known for years how my body was reacting to the cancer and now, I know I am at the end of my life. I am not angry any more in fact most of the time I am relaxed and peaceful but don't waste money on wheelchairs and booking trips for me as I am not going to be able to use either.

4) I don't think I will be going on for much longer and need to tell you how much I love you and to hope the pain and distress of the last four years has not been all bad and that you will remember all of the good times and when I look back we have had a lot of good times the cruises, caravan breaks and the projects we have carried out and for me the pleasure of owning a fleet of brilliant cars. I want you to move on when I have gone and find happiness because you could have forty years without me but given the chance I would do it again because the 11 years has given me all I could ask for.

5) Anyway, back to now I am in almost constant pain when I try to move around and I only get relief when I am lying down. My eyesight is now becoming a problem and is fuzzy a lot of the time. I know you are struggling with our predicament and that it's much harder for you being

left to sort out all the issues. But I don't want a constant stream of visitors or babysitters. If I could talk it would be different but I can't cope.

6) My kids worry me they are obviously distressed and upset but I can't talk to them ether and I would be grateful if you would keep telling them they are welcome, but I am not talking very well.

7) Please don't think badly of me but I want to die, I can't take much more pain and suffering and even being able to go in a wheelchair or the car is no good to me. I am an active man who has lost everything my love life, my working life, my social life, my DIY and now my mobility and ability to communicate, even writing a book is a big problem as I can't stay awake and have to constantly review the chapters.

8) So, if you need me to, I will go in to a hospice or you can arrange respite I will understand. On a few occasions lately you have inferred that the oxygen is not needed and that I carry it everywhere with me, yes, I do because without it I struggle to breath. I did try last night and on Sunday night to leave it off my face, but I wake up with shortage of breath and with all the other issues I have, it's a battle I can do without.

9) We need a better system for medication at night you can't keep running around for morphine and water etc. and then get up and go to work.

It is now the 10th August; we have been struggling with Morphine control over the last few weeks and are now at 300 mg twice per day with top ups as required of Oramorph. This has helped and after a very slow start today I am having a go at the book again.

Sixty Five and Still Alive?

CHAPTER EIGHT

ONCOLOGISTS AND A THORACIC SPECIALIST INPUT

Since the process started in mid-2007 Yvonne and I have diarised every visit to Doctors, Specialists, Healthcare professionals and any visit connected with my illness. This chapter should be used in conjunction with the other chapters to follow the medical milestones and achievements gained over the 4 years. It has been written as a diary starting in 2007 and running forwards to 2011, the X-rays are mine and have been dropped into the book to show the results of various treatments.

24 July 2007 I was admitted to Redditch Alexandra Hospital with suspected pneumonia (a referral from my GP), after an ultrasound and a CT scan it was decided that I had a bad infection of the right lung, I was told it would be possible to treat the infection with drugs in Redditch but it would be better to surgically remove the infection with microsurgery at Heartlands Hospital. Having agreed to a surgical solution I was transferred to Heartlands on the 29th July 2007, X-Rays, scans and more tests took us to the 1st August 2007 the day of my operation.

I went down for surgery at 11am and was told by Yvonne that I was returned to the recovery ward at 5.00pm having had 5 hours in surgery, so when the surgeon came to give me a debrief, I was still thinking micro surgery.

However, the debriefing was positive, the surgeon said the infection was very messy and had been difficult to remove but he had seen nothing sinister, he also said he had sent samples for histology.

The next 10 days were a frustrated recovery from surgery as I contracted post-operative oedema; this is where you swell up like the Michelin man and it took days to go down.

Still the recovery continued and I was told I could be released back home at midday on the 10th August. But even with a discharge notice you had to organise the process yourself. Yvonne arrived at around midday and was shocked to find I had no medication and no release papers available. So off she went to arrange all the relevant documentation.

Sixty Five and Still Alive?

We arrived back home at 4.30pm on the 10th August 2007 after a 4-hour struggle and this was to be the start of my new life.

For the next few days I felt very weak and very unsafe, is unsafe the correct word? Yes, I do mean unsafe I had breathing difficulty, panic attacks and a general feeling of difficulty in getting through the days. Yvonne took me to Kidderminster A&E, referred from NHS Direct. The Doctor on duty referred me to Worcester Royal were I met Professor Lewis for the first time. He listened to me rambling and then said "measure your progress by the week not by the day or by the hour", advice I have followed for four years and advice I have recommended to you in the front of this book.

After an X- ray and tests I was sent home feeling much better; not knowing I had just met a man who was to have great impact on me for the next four years.

I had mentioned in a previous chapter that great emphasis is placed on establishing blame and claiming for injury. Sadly, I fail to be covered by any of the criteria but have made note of my meetings and attempts to claim in Chapter Three so that you can see the lengths you are expected to go to establish blame.

The 17th October has been covered fully in Chapter 2 of this book as has the visits to my doctor on the 18th & 19th October.

My next contact with the medical fraternity was my visit to Redditch Alexandra Hospital to see Jo Hamilton on 7th November 2007. She reviewed my notes and told us there was a lot of thickening on the right-hand side of my lung, the cancer is not curable but she will be there to help with the quality of my life.

Mesothelioma tracks through the scar tissue, so she decided to apply radiotherapy to the scar, normally this is done 1 month after the operation, but due to the loss of the notes relating to my histology we were now 3 months down the line.

The cancer I have is of the type known as Epithelioid, which is the slowest growing of the three types of Mesothelioma. She informed us also that there is a new cancer drug for Mesothelioma called Alimta, which I covered fully in chapter 4.

Sixty Five and Still Alive?

On 15th November we had our first planning meeting for radiotherapy. On 16th November we had an appointment at Heartlands hospital to review progress after the operation. We were told the pleural lining had been taken away, so the lung is now up against the chest wall and they didn't think it necessary to do a full major operation, by removing the lung. The doctor had said he had seen people live up to 7 years after their diagnosis; better than 6 months, I guess. Radiotherapy was carried out over the scheduled two dates on 29th November and the 6th December in Heartlands with a few issues as described in chapter 2.

A meeting was held with the oncology doctor to follow up on the radiotherapy on the 15th January 2008. It was agreed that no more appointments would be booked but we would call her secretary if we noticed any changes, such as shortness of breath, pain, discomfort, cough or weight loss and so we went off to enjoy our life.

We had a number of holidays throughout 2008 and I felt very well. We had a number of good breaks and weekends away but during part of the year I had experienced shortness of breath and difficulty with my lungs that I had put down to a chest infection. In January 2009 we had taken a week in Gran Canaria but I had to be put on the air craft on a lift to return home.

On returning home we made an appointment at our GP's surgery. We went for the appointment with the GP on 3rd February 2009 who referred me straight to the Alexandra Hospital where I was admitted with a suspected chest infection. An X-ray was carried out, showing white area on the right lung. A needle was inserted to try and take fluid off from around the lung, but none was found, so an ultrasound was carried out the next day which identified only pockets of fluid found, so I was discharged with a chest infection and an appointment booked for a CT scan on 11th February 2009.

After the CT scan a visit to the oncologist was attended on 17th February 2009. The scan looked better than the X-ray taken 2 weeks earlier, therefore there was infection there, but she was not sure how much is infection and how much is cancer. The oncologist was to meet with the specialist the next day to review the case and an appointment was booked with the doctor for 5 weeks' time.

Sixty Five and Still Alive?

The X-ray was carried out 11th March 2009 and the results were a lot worse than the one from 3rd February 2009 so the Oncology doctor thinks it is the cancer growing back. Chemotherapy was discussed and agreed to it being carried out. I was given a prescription for steroids and antibiotics and a meeting booked for planning the treatment.

A planning meeting was carried out on 13th March 2009 at the Garden suite explaining the process of chemotherapy and outcome.

18/3/09: My first chemotherapy session was given at the Garden Suite, Redditch. Oncologists review, on 29th March 2009, of the X-ray shows the top of lung can now be seen, but the doctor still thinks there is an infection, so three weeks of antibiotics were given.

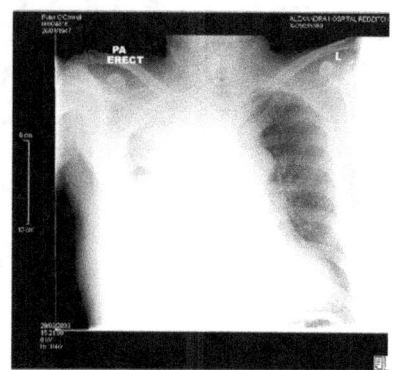

30/3/09: Appointment with GP and asked about a referral to see Dr Lewis at Worcester. The Macmillan Nurse then visited us for the first time on 1st April 2009, Alison, a nice nurse who helped with medication for sputum that I was coughing up.

Chemotherapy was due to be given three weekly as long as the blood results are OK. The chemotherapy consisted of two drugs Alimta and Carboplatin. Alimta is the drug used for Mesothelioma and Carboplatin is for non-small cell lung cancer. The infusion took around two hours for both drugs.

We had another appt with Dr Hamilton on 7th April 2009 and said, "it is the cancer and if the chemo doesn't work then you will have 3-4 weeks left". The blood results done for the second chemo were not good enough to have dose number two, so this was delayed for a week until 15th April 2009.

The next appointment was on 29th April 2009 to have blood samples taken. The results showed low platelets and blood count. Two units of blood were given; therefore, the chemo was delayed for another week.

Sixty Five and Still Alive?

The 3rd chemo dose was given on 6th May 2009 and by this time I was feeling much better and I gave the nebuliser back on 15th May 2009.

On 17th May 2009 we visited Coventry ward 35, as I found it difficult to move around I had a blood test, it was found the red blood count to be low, another blood test was taken on 18th May 2009, when it was decided that 2 more units of blood should be given. During the transfusion I noticed a rash that had developed on my skin and the doctor said it was shingles! I was given some tablets to take.

Our three-weekly appointment with the oncologist on 26th May 2009 took place, but even though the shingles was better, it was decided to leave the chemo number 4 for another week. Chemo number 4 was given on 3rd June 2009 and we went for our appointment with Prof Lewis on 11/6/09. An X-ray was taken, and it was the best results he had ever seen with chemotherapy and the breathing tests were back to 2 years ago.

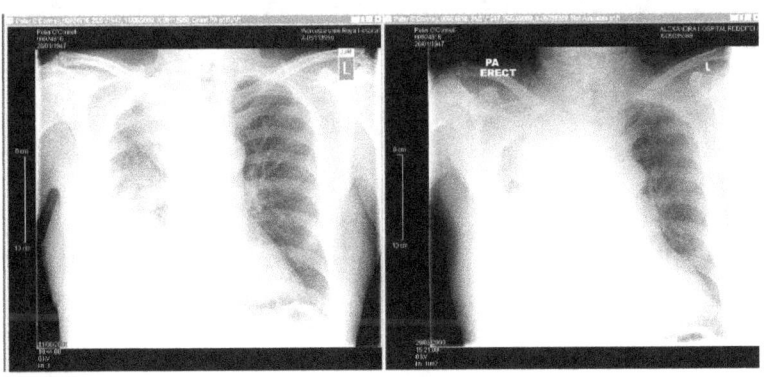

X-ray taken 11/6/09   *X-ray taken 29/3/09*

14/6/09: Having felt OK I went to stay in a premier travel inn, as I had a job to do the next day. When I woke up in the morning, it looked like a blood bath! I had had a bad nosebleed; blood was all over the sheets & pillowcases. Sorry - Premier Inns. So yet again more platelets and blood transfusions. Yet another delay on chemo number 5.

Sixty Five and Still Alive?

Chemo 5 was eventually given on 1st July 2009, then 13th July another unit of platelets and on 21st July, two more units of blood. It was then agreed due to the harm the chemo was doing to my bone marrow, that the chemo should be stopped.

The next appointment was with Prof Lewis on 13th August 2009 who had done another X-ray. The results were amazing, he said it was a miracle. Miracles don't usually happen to me. Four inches of tumour had been removed.

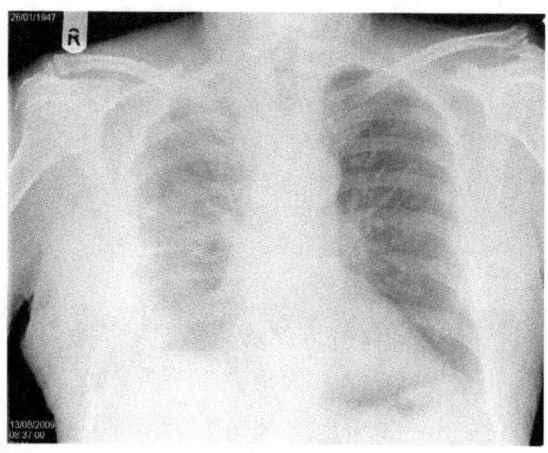

X-ray taken August 2009

The difference from March 2009 to August 2009 was clearly evident.

So off for holidays, visited lots of places in the UK and booked a cruise to the canaries.

The next follow up was on 12th October 2009, where there appeared to be no change to the X-ray from August. Good news again.

Sixty Five and Still Alive?

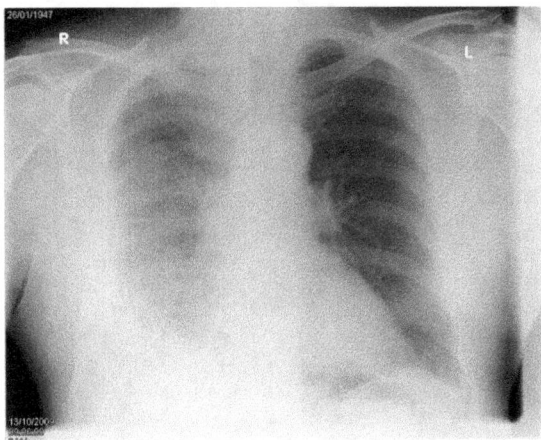

X-ray taken August Oct 2009

Next follow up was on the 26th November 2009 with Prof Lewis, he said the results were better than August. Breathing results has changed from 58 in August to 61 in November.

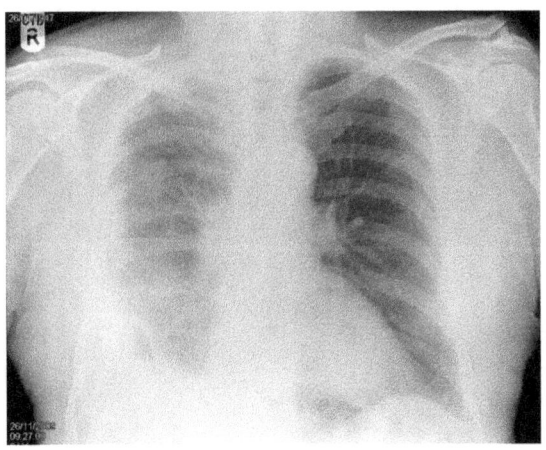

X-ray taken November 2009

Follow ups then on 19th January 2010 & 1st April 2010 showed no change to the X-rays and that the disease was stable at the moment. Weight had gained from 13st 7 in August 2009 to 15st 12 in April 2010, no wonder I had to keep buying more clothes!!

Sixty Five and Still Alive?

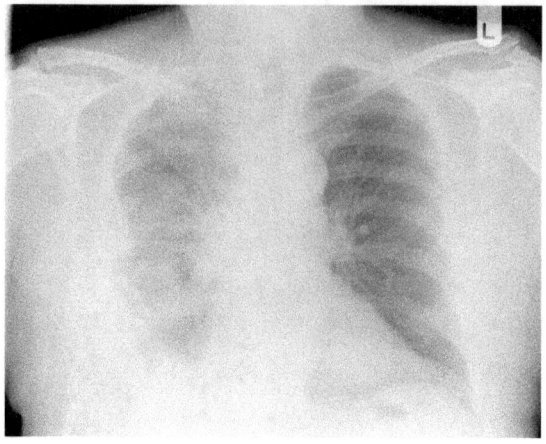

X-ray taken April 2010

In May 2010 we went to the Isle of Wight for a week, and I started with back pain. Once home, I went to see the GP and was given tramadol, but the pain just got worse and worse. It was also then painful in the chest and thick catarrh developed, green tea helped to clear for a few minutes, then I found it difficult to talk. Pain became so intense; it was difficult to move around.

Results of a CT scan on 15th June showed that the cancer had gone into the bone, so the oncologist decided to give some radiotherapy to the spine, to avoid the cancer pressing on the spinal column. 20 gray over 5 fractions were delivered, starting on 17th June. I was also given Oramorph to help with the pain, but due to the amount I was taking, I was put on MST tablets too.

27/6/10: We went away on a caravan holiday to Wales, we have a tourer which I helped push out of the drive. I drove to Wales and during the week found I had bad pain in my arm. I visited the doctors to be told it could be from the radiotherapy, so I took some morphine. On Thursday it was not better, so visited Bangor Hospital to be told the same thing. They gave me some steroids to help. By Saturday morning, we went back to the hospital, this time I insisted on an X-ray and found that my humorous was broken straight across my arm! No wonder I had been in agony, they strapped it up and sent me away.

On returning home on the 5th July I went to A & E, who made me an appointment for the fracture clinic on the Tuesday. They felt the fracture was

Sixty Five and Still Alive?

due to cancer in the bone, the oncologist was contacted and it was agreed I should have the arm pinned.

I was booked in on Saturday 10th July, an X-ray was taken but as it was worse than 1st April 2010 there were many conversations regarding the anaesthetic and nerve block, however they went ahead with the operation with no nerve block. Operation conducted at 12 noon.

The X-rays below look like something out of Frankenstein!

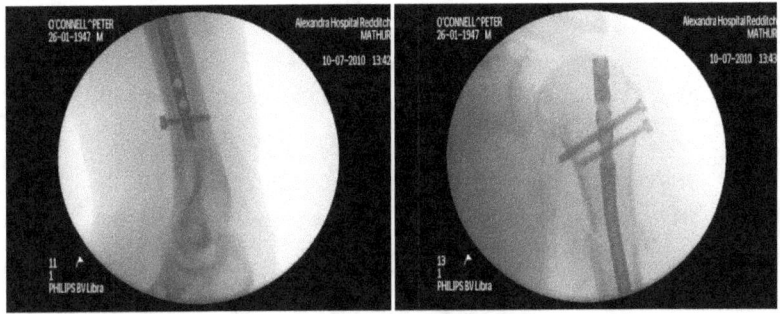

Discharged the next day, with a radiotherapy appointment booked for 4th August 2010, as mesothelioma tracks through the scar tissue, this was to prevent this. Physiotherapy was then started.

On 28th July I felt feverish and went to my GP who said I may have an infection, so issued me with Amoxicillin, then on a visit to the A & E on the 29th, due to bad pain in my arm, I was told this was normal after pinning and sent me home.

On Monday 2nd August 2010, I went to an appointment with the physiotherapist who looked at my shoulder as the top of my arm was swollen; he passed me straight to the bone specialist, who booked me into the Alexandra Hospital for an operation to clean out the infection. Operation was at 3pm. I was kept in with the wound open and given IV antibiotics, then another operation on 4th August 2010 to clean and stitch the wound. Discharged on the 5th having missed my appointment at the Walsgrave Hospital for radiotherapy. A meeting with the oncologist on the 11th rebooked the radiotherapy for 19th August 2010. She also suggested that we do some more chemo as my breathing was getting worse too.

Sixty Five and Still Alive?

1st dose of chemo was given on 15th September 2010, I was fine at first until day 7 when I began to get very tired, by day 10 I had a rash that was very itchy and on speaking to the Garden Suite, they reckon I had an allergic reaction to the chemo, so antihistamine tablets were taken.

At the next appointment with the oncologist doctor on 29th September, she agreed it was an allergic reaction to the chemo and she suggested we could stop if I wanted to but as it was so effective last year I decided to go on with the next dose, but at a reduced amount similar to that given to me last year.

2nd dose of chemo was given on 6th October after the normal blood tests which were OK for the next dose, even though the red blood cells were only 10. Nose started bleeding on 10th October, but no rash, it was decided that the rash on the first dose was from Codine Phosphate (a pain killer I had been taking).

We went back to Worcester to see Prof Lewis on 7th October and he was very upbeat and told me that the X-ray showed the chemo is working again and the arm was healing.

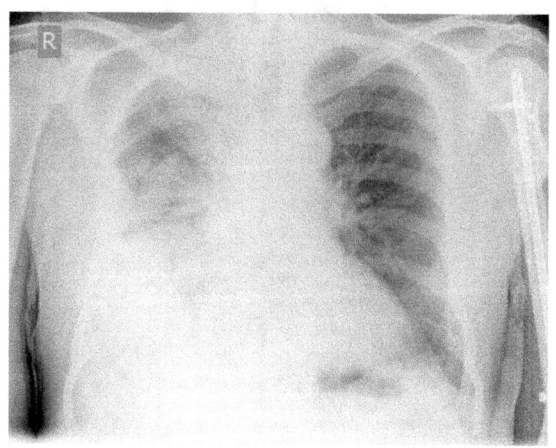

X-ray taken October 2010

The bone doctors I saw on 15th October 2010, discharged me and explained that there was no cancer in the arm otherwise it would not have healed. It had healed very well around the pin.

Sixty Five and Still Alive?

Blood tests were taken on 15th October 2010 and the results were not good, Platelets 26, red cells 8.8 and low white cells, so 2 units of blood and 2 units of platelets given. Thanks to all these donors.

A week later I was feeling ill and was admitted to the Alexandra Hospital as I had a cold, they gave me some antibiotics and discharged the next day.

After the next appointment with the oncologist we agreed we should carry on with a 3rd dose but also have a CT scan on 15th November.

3rd dose of chemo was given on 27th October. I was starting to feel worse as we got to the 4th November, so went for some blood tests, but the results were not low enough to do any transfusions. The weekend was the worst I had had in a while, no energy and sleeping all the time, by Monday more bloods were taken showing NO white blood cells, 7 platelets and an 8 red blood count. My blood system was on the floor! Two units of blood and one of platelets were given immediately and I was told I should have gone to A & E over the weekend, but I didn't want to sit in a comprised situation for four hours and the A & E is a very drafty place. More tests on the 11th were still not good so two more units of blood and one of platelets were given.

Next meeting with the oncologist, she was very upset and said I could have died when my blood system was on the floor and I should have gone to A & E. Considered myself told off. We decided to stop chemo.

Various blood tests over the next few weeks showed they were returning to normal.

Hope you are still with me, now to my final year 2011.

Over Christmas I couldn't resist doing DIY, we had started the change round of the office into the bedroom and I needed to get on with it, but by January I had bad pain in my chest, so we visited the oncologist on 4th January 2011. She said the pain was lower than the cancer I had in my sternum picked up from a CT scan, so I carried on with the pain killers.

Another appointment with Prof Lewis and more good news the X-ray carried out showed the chest back to how it was in November 2009. Chemo had worked well again; it was worth the trauma.

Sixty Five and Still Alive?

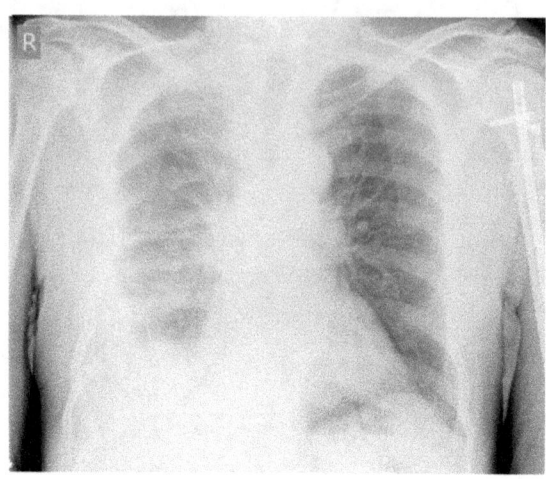

X-ray taken January 2011

The pain in my chest was still bad so I was given some inflammatory tablets to take.

The good news allowed us to book another cruise to the Mediterranean for my 64th birthday on 26th Jan, however on 20th January 2011, I was walking the dog on the beach and felt that I had hurt my back. I had a couple of appointments with an osteopath, before we went on the cruise, but this did not help much. I spent most of the time on the ship in my cabin lying down as I could not sit up or move about without serious pain. I spent a fortune on acupuncture & massages to try and get rid of the pain, but nothing helped. Once back in the UK we went straight to A & E who took an X-ray and suggested we see the oncologist. The meeting on 8th March 2011 was not the best we had had, as the oncologist said to Yvonne and I that I may not make it to Christmas, how right she was. She arranged for radiotherapy to the spine which was delivered on 21st March 2011.

Sixty Five and Still Alive?

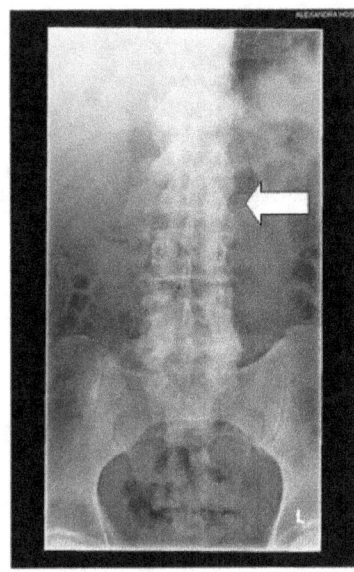 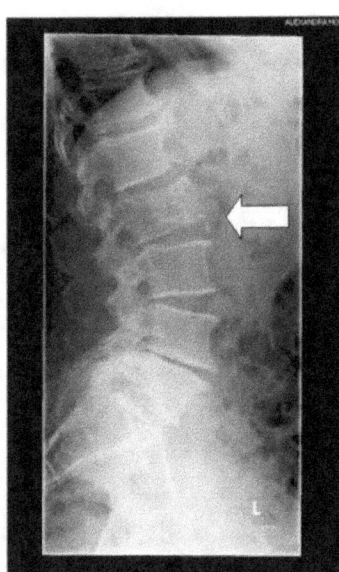

You can see from above the 4 vertebra up from the bottom was distorted due to the cancer in my spine.

Over the last few months I had begun to get a lump on my shoulder on the scar tissue from the pin I had in my arm last year, mesothelioma tracks through the scar tissue. We had our next appointment with Prof Lewis on 7th April 2011, who said he would ask the oncologist if she would do some more radiotherapy to the lump, he also arranged a bone scan which was done on 28th April. An X-ray carried out showed little change.

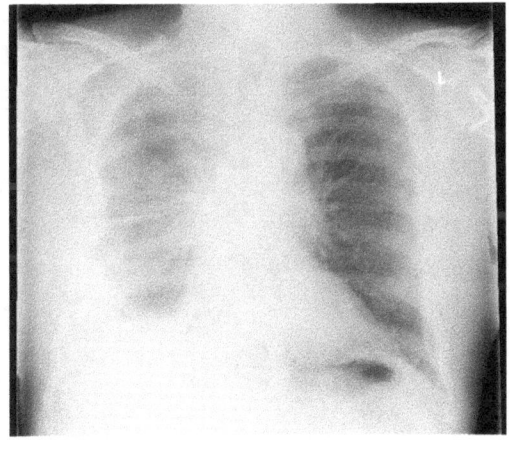

At a meeting with the oncologist on 19th April, she agreed to do radiotherapy on the lump but was not sure if would help as it had already been done after the operation, but I insisted we did. This was carried out on 11th May. We discussed

Sixty Five and Still Alive?

more chemo, but this was no longer an option due to the reaction during the last round. I also got thrush again in my mouth so was prescribed for that too. She also suggested taking 30 mgs of MST tablets (morphine slow release) to help with the pain.

The results of the bone scan were discussed with Prof Lewis on 19th May 2011, there appears to be black spots (cancer) in the following areas.

1. Bottom of left arm – elbow
2. One in pelvis
3. Top of right leg
4. Sternum
5. Right clavicle
6. Couple in the spine

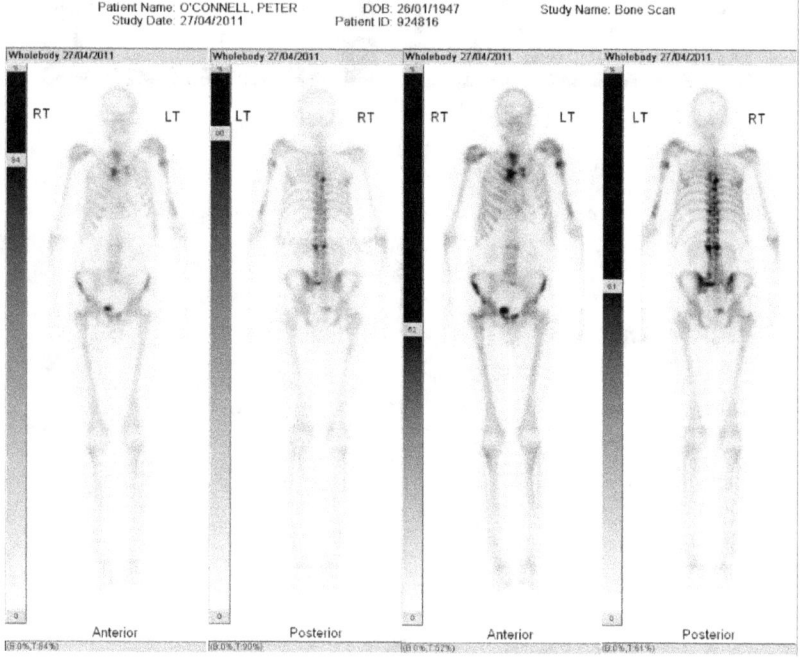

Blood tests taken also showed the folic acid to be low, so tablets were given by the GP for a month.

Sixty Five and Still Alive?

The Macmillan Nurses who had been visiting on and off throughout my illness then started to play an important role in my care.

The pain started to get worse and MST tablets were increased on 15th June 2011 to 90mgs. A lovely lady doctor from the hospice visited who suggested I also took Ibuprofen tablets 4 times a day as this was good for bone pain. On 21st June our GP increased this to 100 mgs as I had drunk a bottle of Oramorph (liquid morphine) in a week.

A meeting on the 23rd June with the oncologist said there was no point in doing any more radiotherapy as it would not help with the cancer and painkillers are the best option but would consider an MRI scan which was booked for 1st July.

I woke up on the 30th June with my left arm (the one with the pin in it) all swollen up, so we tripped down to A & E, where they tried to take some fluid, but nothing much came. They kept me in on IV antibiotics and after various tests decided my lymph system had packed up due to the cancer. The oncologist came to see me and we asked her how long I had got left, she said 2 – 3 months. She was right again.

I was discharged on the 7th July 2011

From then on it was a downward spiral. Morphine increased on a regular basis and I lost over a stone in weight in a month. The Macmillan nurses visited every week and by 16th August I was taking 400mgs twice a day of MST with regular Oramorph top ups.

I stopped eating on Friday 19th August 2011, I only managed a half of bacon and tomato sandwich in the morning and I couldn't face anything else after this. That day the Vicar, (Ric the Vic), came to see me as I had asked for him to carry out my service at the funeral, we prepared the service and picked the hymns and music.

I was quite aware of my surroundings and not too high on the morphine, however things changed for the worse in the early hours of Monday 22nd August. I was sick with bile, all over the floor, so Yvonne called out the district nurses. They gave me an injection, to help with the nausea and asked Yvonne to try and get my oral MST tablets (which were now 600 mgs twice a day) down me in the morning. I got one tablet down, but the next one I was sick again. So at 7am I had another visit by the nursing staff and another injection for the sickness including a morphine injection for the pain. Another bout of sickness

Sixty Five and Still Alive?

again at 12 noon and yet another injection from the nurses. From then they then decided to put me on a syringe driver, so they could have a constant flow of drugs into me to help with the sickness and pain.

After the driver was inserted at 3.30pm, I was in and out of sleep getting agitated and not generally knowing what was going on. Yvonne tells me I didn't sleep much that night and kept having hallucinations and very agitated trying to pull my oxygen pipe about.

My last day Tuesday 23rd August, Michelle's Birthday. There was a stream of visitors to the house. The vicar popped in again, the Macmillan nurse came and arranged a bed bath for me, pity I wasn't well enough to notice the nice ladies ☺ , a care man came to arrange a care plan for the coming days, I had various doses of drugs to help me sleep but none had much effect until the dose at 3.30pm when the syringe driver was changed. From then on, I was in a deep sleep. My son and daughter turned up at 4.30pm and from this time, a noise like a restriction in my throat was heard. At 6pm Yvonne, Kay and Neil tried to sit me up to help with my breathing, and this is when I woke to find my son, and a big cuddle we had.

From then I don't remember anything more. Our GP called round at 7.30pm to see me and gave me an injection to help with the rattle noise and said to Yvonne, Kay and Neil that I had only a few hours left.

My family were with me at the end and it was a peaceful passing. I had wanted to go for some months as the pain was bad, now I was gone and out of pain, in my favourite bed and new bedroom. Just as I had wanted.

I passed away on 23rd August 2011 at 9.20pm and was certified by the district nurses at 9.30pm. The funeral directors collected me at 12.40am.

On 24th August 2011 the doctors phoned Yvonne to explain the process of obtaining a death certificate and the need to call the Coroner. The Coroner phoned and decided no post-mortem was required as samples were taken from me at the operation in 2007 and there was no doubt it was Mesothelioma; however, an inquest will be heard on 18th October 2011.

The funeral was booked for 2pm on the 2nd September 2011 at Redditch Crematorium.

Sixty Five and Still Alive?

It was just as I had wanted, horses and carriage, my hymns and music and over 100 people, with standing room for some. My Eulogy was read out, that I had written in my last month. You did a great job Marie. A lovely day to remember me by.

Sixty Five and Still Alive?

EULOGY

Peter O'Connell

26/01/1947 - 23/08/2011

Well I would think if you are listening to this eulogy I am not around anymore, and in terms of DIY this address has been my last project.

A few months ago, I attended Albert Rodgers funeral.

Albert is Yvonne's Dad; I found the address to be excellent as the speaker Reverend Purdy knew him very well both from a business relationship and in later years as a friend. So, his words matched the man and the occasion.

I have no such friendships with orators or people who have ecclesiastical expertise, so I promised Yvonne I would take it on as my last DIY job.

The finished version to be read at my funeral, by whoever feels they could take on the challenge. Thank you, Marie, for feeling you could take on the job L.O.L

In 2007 my life changed when I was diagnosed with Mesothelioma, as most of you will know this cancer is asbestos related and is incurable and I have no Idea where it came from but I sure know what it does in terms of destruction and devastation when you have it.

So, what has happened to me over the last 64 years?

I was born in Birmingham on the 26 January 1947 and grew up as an only child in and around the Birmingham area, ending this phase of my life here in Bromsgrove. Both my parents were only children to which is why it's probably very empty in here and you have plenty of room to sit down.

I have experienced much happiness in my life, sometimes tinged with a little sadness but I have no regrets, who could have regrets when they have a wonderful wife, children who love them and grandchildren who show genuine love and compassion and with me I have also had the privilege and pleasure of two extended families who have more than made up for my own lack of siblings, my dad told me if you had achieved perfection stop.

Sixty Five and Still Alive?

But I am not sure he is right because both of my kids are perfect, but we really would be struggling for people in here today if I had listened to him.

I have had two marriages that have helped to shape the last 40 years and of course the input into my formative years from my parents.

My life has brought me success and good reward to effort in terms of lifestyle, but as restarts we are not well off.

I have sat and reflected on my 64 years on this earth and I felt I needed to put something back in to the process of cancer research and treatment so I have attempted to write a book on Mesothelioma that cover my trials and tribulations with the illness and have asked that the proceeds are given to Macmillan Cancer Support and Cancer Research for Mesothelioma project work

The small impact that Mesothelioma has across the world means it will never receive funding commensurate with the suffering it creates so I decided to put my own effort in to its support.

Religion has never played a large part in my life, but I do believe that we should all do everything we can to help others while they are alive and I have tried to live this way.

Kay you are a wonderful Daughter and you have shown amassing love and compassion to me over the last few years, the grand kids have also added a lot to my life in terms of happiness. I know you will have many happy years ahead of you with Adrian and the girls so chill and enjoy life and Kay J F D I.

Neil, as my only son your always on my mind. I would have liked to see you settled down but to have seen your happiness over the last few years with Bea has been good and I am sure your future will bring you happiness, you have a loving nature and deserve to be loved in return.

I was married to Val for 33 years, who like Yvonne helped me and assisted me in everything I did and she gave me two wonderful children and the happy memories and successes of my younger years.

Yvonne life can be very cruel when an illness contracted decades ago can shorten life by 20/30 years, we only managed 13 years or so together, but I would not change them for anything.

We found something together that I *think* is very rare.

Sixty Five and Still Alive?

We found love but also "trust, truth and how to be happy just being together" without the need to buy things or to keep running off spending money, this is what I think true love is, but now you need to go and fulfil our dreams that we didn't manage to complete together for me.

Today is not for sadness as I am now at peace, which is a place I have needed to be for a long time, Mesothelioma is painful and debilitating when it moves in to the bone and now it is now my turn to rest from the constant pain and distress I have been experiencing for months and months.

Over the last few years I have fought this cancer that has now claimed my life as most of you know I wanted to live for three score years and ten, but this was not meant to be.

I think this illness has made me a better person and taught me patience and gave me a calmer outlook on life but it would have been good to have had a few more years.

So, I will no longer have any input in to your day to day lives but please carry with you, my love, affection and support for the rest of your lives and remember me kindly as someone who cares for you deeply

God bless you all

Pete.

Sixty Five and Still Alive?

CHAPTER NINE

HOW SHOULD I PREPARE MYSELF FOR THE END OF LIFE?

This is not a subject I have spent any time thinking or worrying about but it does need to be addressed; I genuinely don't know how I feel now that my death is inevitable and I must accept three years longer than the average life expectancy from diagnosis to death is what I will have achieved making around four years in total.

I have had some great holidays; I have managed to work and earn money through most of the illness which has helped fund our life style and the O'Connell fleet of brilliant vehicles. During my illness I have met and spent time with lots of super people both sufferers, medics and carers.

Talking to people on how to be a survivor is easy, telling the kids the end is nigh is quite a different issue. I have started to write letters to Yvonne telling her how I feel and have now got over the worst of my issues, as everyone becomes aware of the way I feel and what I need. I can talk to people rationally on what I want and when I want it; so my advice is: do what you feel best with.

So writing notes is one way, the Macmillan nurses are excellent source of information and will help at every opportunity, but for me I looked back over the last four years and I am no longer angry. I have had years to put things in order so that I don't have to worry, but I still have been able to work and play most of the time and I believe that I have gained much from the people and processes this illness has brought me in contact with. I have learnt that 'my cup is half full' is the same as 'my cup is half empty' but when a medical professional tells you something, 'the cup being half full' is a better way to hear it. I have learnt that the NHS is very good at delivering treatment and cures but is dreadful at looking after me when admitted as a patient. But is that me, is it how I deal with the situations?

Sixty Five and Still Alive?

CHAPTER TEN

COUNSELLING WORDS OF WISDOM AND ALL THAT

Since leaving the Alexandra Hospital in May/June 2011. I have been thinking about the end of life, the end of my life and it is a very sobering process. I have lived for sixty-four years and like most people have little to show for it. We have material belongings, reduced by two divorces.

I have two kids and Yvonne has two kids and I have currently got two grandchildren, this figure will rise as time passes and the younger ones settle down, but no real impact will be left by my passing and I find that a sad reflection. So, I hope that this short story and my attempts to share my thoughts and fears with you, during what for me, has been the most serious and significant event in my life - Mesothelioma.

A whole raft of help and advice has been made available, but I have refused most of it. Why have I refused this help and advice, well in the early stages I was very angry and did not want to accept the diagnosis.

Then as time went by, I was getting conflicting information so decided to wait till the end. As the end arrived, I think fear has moved in and said "play it by ear, just play it by ear." It is now August 2011 and I wake up in the early hours thinking "not yet then?"

I have a weekly visit from a Macmillan nursing team, a twice a month visit from a district nurse and a phone line to my GP for Yvonne to call and order medication and get help. To date we have had two visits from the Doctor and the system seems to be working.

I decided to die at home with my wife and familiar surroundings, I hope we can achieve this as I love my home and surroundings and have found the time in hospital distressing; Yvonne is probably the worst nurse you could ever find but she is my nurse and she cares for me.

As I get weaker our problems will increase but we will cope. We have now, on the 10th August 2011, arranged to have help from the local hospice (a three-day sit in service) that will let Yvonne go to work and see how that goes.

CHAPTER ELEVEN

LIFE WITHOUT PETE

As you may have guessed I had to finish the last of the book for Pete, as during the last week he was obviously not capable.

It's early days since the funeral but my life is now empty, I constantly cry, something I have never done in my life, I can't even write this without tears rolling down my face.

I walk into our lovely bedroom and expect to see him there, I lie in bed at night and hold my hand out to hold his, but he is not there. His chair in the lounge is empty now.

I have loads of flowers around the house from the funeral, I did not want to leave them behind at the crematorium and Pete will be reunited with them soon, once I bring his ashes back. The smell is fantastic and a reminder of the day which Pete planned and worked out to be just perfect, a name I used to call him at BSI - Peter Perfect!

My daughters have been great and I wish to thank Marie and her family for the help and support they too have given me.

Pete and I did everything together and I miss him already, just popping out to the shops on my own is very odd. I have not gone back to work yet, but will try a half day tomorrow, 9th September 2011. I can hear Pete saying, "you need the money go to work!"

As Pete said, the last 11 years have been the best I could have wished for and I have some lovely memories. We had some fantastic holidays and cruises and some great photos for me to remember him by. A nice fleet of cars, but I do need to sell one of them, three cars for me is a bit excessive! I will keep the touring caravan and have booked on a manoeuvring course, for some practice. Pete use to do all the driving while towing. The house is a constant reminder of all his DIY; let's hope he trained me well with the brownie badges I have collected, so I can keep it from falling down!

Sixty Five and Still Alive?

So, I will try and carry on like you wanted Pete and visit the Panama Canal and Alaska, that we didn't do off your wish list. Time, I hope, will be a great healer, but I will never forget you. Thanks for a wonderful time.

I know you are at peace now, out of all the constant pain you had, I just wish we could have had longer together, life can be so cruel.

I hope you all have enjoyed this book and it helps others to battle against this disease. Never give up and Vic, get as much out of life as possible.

As Pete wanted, the proceeds from the sale of this book are to go to Macmillan Cancer Support and Cancer Research for the continuing investigation into Mesothelioma and how to cure and support this dreadful disease.

Take Care.

Sixty Five and Still Alive?

BIBLIOGRAPHY

http://www.solutionsdoc.co.uk/documents/OVERBREATHING.pdf

http://www.reiki.org/faq/whatisreiki.html

http://www.reflexology-research.com/whatis.htm

http://www.ukskeptics.com/acupuncture.php

All last accessed 16/9/11